CONTENTS

INTRODUCTION

In a world where fad diets come and go, there is one timeless approach to eating that stands out for its holistic benefits and delectable flavors—the Mediterranean diet. Rooted in the rich cultural heritage of the Mediterranean region, this way of nourishing the body has captivated the taste buds and hearts of countless individuals for centuries. From the sun-kissed coastlines of Greece and Italy to the vibrant markets of Morocco and Spain, the Mediterranean diet embodies the essence of balance, simplicity, and sheer culinary delight.

This book is an invitation to embark on a gastronomic journey, exploring the abundant gifts bestowed upon us by the Mediterranean. Beyond being a mere diet, it is a lifestyle —an embodiment of the values held dear by those who savor life's pleasures, relish communal meals, and embrace the wisdom of generations past. It offers a beacon of hope in an era when processed foods and fast-paced living have taken a toll on our well-being.

The Mediterranean diet is a beautiful tapestry of fresh

fruits and vegetables, hearty whole grains, aromatic herbs and spices, lean proteins, and the crown jewel of its cuisine—the golden elixir known as olive oil. It showcases the symphony of colors and flavors found in nature's bounty, harmonizing together to create nourishing and mouthwatering dishes. But more than just a delightful culinary experience, the Mediterranean diet has been widely praised by researchers and health professionals for its numerous health benefits.

Studies have shown that adhering to the Mediterranean diet can reduce the risk of chronic diseases such as heart disease, stroke, and certain types of cancer. Its emphasis on plant-based foods, healthy fats, and moderate portions provides a blueprint for maintaining a healthy weight, improving cardiovascular health, and promoting longevity. Furthermore, this way of eating has been linked to cognitive benefits, protecting against age-related mental decline and fostering a sharper mind.

Beyond the physical aspects, the Mediterranean diet celebrates the art of savoring each meal and cherishing the company of loved ones around the table. It reminds us to slow down, to appreciate the sensory journey of food, and to create a sense of community through shared meals. In a world driven by instant gratification, the Mediterranean diet beckons us to reconnect with the timeless rituals of mindful eating and meaningful connections.

Throughout the pages of this book, we will delve into the foundations of the Mediterranean diet, explore its key components, and provide practical guidance on incorporating its principles into your daily life. From simple and nourishing recipes to practical tips for grocery shopping and meal planning, we will empower you to embrace the Mediterranean lifestyle and unlock its transformative benefits.

So, whether you seek a path to vibrant health, culinary inspiration, or a deeper appreciation for the simple pleasures of life, join us on this journey to discover the captivating world of the Mediterranean diet. Together, let us embrace the sun-soaked flavors, celebrate the joy of wholesome eating, and embark on a life-changing adventure that nourishes both body and soul.

CHAPTER ONE

Introduction

a. Overview of the Mediterranean Diet

The Mediterranean Diet is a widely acclaimed dietary pattern inspired by the eating habits of people living in countries surrounding the Mediterranean Sea, such as Greece, Italy, Spain, and Morocco. It is known for its emphasis on whole foods, fresh produce, lean proteins, and healthy fats. The diet has gained significant popularity in recent years due to its potential health benefits and its ability to promote a well-balanced and sustainable approach to eating.

One of the key characteristics of the Mediterranean Diet is the high consumption of fruits, vegetables, legumes, nuts, and whole grains. These foods provide essential vitamins, minerals, and dietary fiber, contributing to overall health and well-being. Additionally, the diet encourages the consumption of lean proteins like fish, poultry, and legumes, while limiting red meat intake.

Another notable aspect of the Mediterranean Diet is the use of healthy fats, particularly olive oil. Olive oil is a staple in this diet and is rich in monounsaturated fats, which have been associated with reduced risk of heart disease. It is often used as a replacement for other cooking oils and butter.

The Mediterranean Diet is also characterized by moderate consumption of dairy products, such as cheese and yogurt. These provide important nutrients like calcium and probiotics, which support bone health and a healthy gut microbiome. However, it is important to choose low-fat or reduced-fat options to avoid excessive saturated fat intake.

In addition to the food choices, the Mediterranean Diet places an emphasis on mindful and social eating. Meals are typically enjoyed with family and friends, and there is a focus on savoring the flavors and taking time to appreciate the meal. This approach promotes a positive relationship with food and can contribute to improved digestion and satisfaction.

Overall, the Mediterranean Diet offers a well-rounded and flexible approach to nutrition. It encourages a diverse range of foods, which provides a wide array of nutrients necessary for optimal health. The diet's emphasis on whole, unprocessed foods and healthy fats contributes to its potential benefits for heart health, weight management, and chronic disease prevention.

b. Historical and cultural background

The Mediterranean Diet is deeply rooted in the history and culture of the Mediterranean region. Its origins can be traced back thousands of years, with influences from ancient civilizations such as the Greeks and the Romans.

Historically, the Mediterranean region has been a hub of trade and cultural exchange, resulting in a diverse array of culinary traditions. The diet draws inspiration from the agricultural practices and food availability of the region, incorporating ingredients that were abundant and accessible to the Mediterranean population.

The traditional Mediterranean Diet was heavily influenced by the agricultural practices of the time. People relied on locally grown fruits, vegetables, and grains, as well as the bounty of the sea for fish and seafood. Olive trees were cultivated for their oil, and herbs and spices were used to enhance the flavors of dishes.

Furthermore, the Mediterranean Diet has cultural and social significance within the communities that practice it. Mealtimes are often seen as an opportunity for connection and celebration, with an emphasis on shared meals and the enjoyment of food. This cultural aspect reinforces the importance of the Mediterranean Diet as a way of life rather than just a list of dietary guidelines.

c. Benefits of the Mediterranean Diet

The Mediterranean Diet has been extensively studied for its potential health benefits. Numerous research studies have demonstrated that following this dietary pattern can have positive effects on various aspects of health.

- Cardiovascular health: The Mediterranean Diet has been associated with a reduced risk of heart disease and stroke. The high consumption of fruits, vegetables, whole grains, and healthy fats, along with the moderate intake of lean proteins, contributes to improved heart health. The monounsaturated fats in olive oil, in particular, have been shown to lower levels of LDL cholesterol and reduce the risk of heart disease.

- Weight management: The Mediterranean Diet is not a strict calorie-restrictive diet but rather focuses on a balanced and sustainable approach to eating. The emphasis on whole, unprocessed foods and the inclusion of healthy fats and fiber-rich foods can help promote satiety and prevent overeating. Additionally, the diet encourages regular physical activity, which is essential for maintaining a healthy weight.
- Diabetes prevention: Following the Mediterranean Diet has been associated with a lower risk of developing type 2 diabetes. The diet's emphasis on complex carbohydrates from whole grains and legumes, along with the consumption of fruits and vegetables, contributes to improved blood sugar control. The Mediterranean Diet also encourages the consumption of lean proteins, which can help regulate blood sugar levels.
- Anti-inflammatory effects: Chronic inflammation is linked to various health conditions, including heart disease, cancer, and arthritis. The Mediterranean Diet is rich in foods with anti-inflammatory properties, such as fruits, vegetables, olive oil, and fatty fish. These foods contain antioxidants and other bioactive compounds that can help reduce inflammation in the body.
- Cognitive health: Several studies have suggested that the Mediterranean Diet may play a role in maintaining cognitive function and reducing the risk of age-related cognitive decline and neurodegenerative diseases like Alzheimer's disease. The diet's emphasis on antioxidants and

anti-inflammatory foods, along with its potential to improve heart health, may contribute to brain health as well.

In conclusion, the Mediterranean Diet offers a holistic approach to nutrition, drawing inspiration from the rich culinary traditions and cultural practices of the Mediterranean region. Its emphasis on whole, unprocessed foods, healthy fats, and mindful eating has been associated with numerous health benefits, including improved cardiovascular health, weight management, diabetes prevention, and cognitive well-being. By adopting the Mediterranean Diet, individuals can embrace a sustainable and enjoyable way of eating that promotes overall health and vitality.

The Mediterranean Lifestyle

a. Exploring the holistic approach to health

The holistic approach to health recognizes that individuals are not just physical beings but also have mental, emotional, and spiritual aspects that contribute to their overall well-being. It emphasizes the interconnectedness of these different dimensions and aims to promote balance and harmony in all areas of life. By considering the whole person rather than focusing solely on specific symptoms or diseases, the holistic approach seeks to support optimal health and vitality.

Holistic health takes into account various factors that can influence well-being, including diet, exercise, sleep, stress levels, social connections, and environmental factors. It recognizes that these factors are interconnected and that imbalances in one area can affect other aspects of a person's health. Therefore, the goal of the holistic approach is to address these imbalances and promote a state of equilibrium.

One key aspect of the holistic approach is the recognition that the mind and body are closely connected. Mental and emotional well-being can have a significant impact on physical health, and vice versa. Practices such as mindfulness, meditation, and psychotherapy are often utilized to promote emotional balance and reduce stress, which can positively influence physical health.

Furthermore, the holistic approach acknowledges the importance of prevention and maintaining wellness, rather than solely focusing on treating diseases. It encourages individuals to take an active role in their health by adopting healthy lifestyle habits, such as eating nutritious foods, engaging in regular physical activity, managing stress, and getting sufficient rest.

b. Physical activity and its importance

Physical activity plays a crucial role in maintaining overall health and well-being. Regular exercise has numerous benefits for the body, mind, and even emotional state. Engaging in physical activity helps strengthen muscles, improves cardiovascular health, enhances flexibility and mobility, and supports healthy weight management.

One of the primary benefits of physical activity is its positive impact on cardiovascular health. Regular exercise helps strengthen the heart and improves blood circulation, reducing the risk of heart disease, high blood pressure, and stroke. It also increases the levels of HDL cholesterol (the "good" cholesterol) while reducing levels of LDL cholesterol (the "bad" cholesterol).

Physical activity is also essential for maintaining a healthy weight. Engaging in regular exercise helps burn calories, increase metabolism, and build lean muscle mass. It can aid in weight loss or weight maintenance and reduce the risk of obesity-related conditions such as type 2 diabetes and certain types of cancer.

In addition to its physical benefits, exercise has a profound impact on mental and emotional well-being. It promotes the release of endorphins, often referred to as "feel-good" hormones, which can boost mood, reduce stress, and alleviate symptoms of depression and anxiety. Regular physical activity is also associated with improved cognitive function and better sleep quality.

It's important to note that physical activity encompasses a broad range of activities and can be tailored to individual preferences and abilities. It can include aerobic exercises like walking, running, swimming, or cycling, as well as strength training, flexibility exercises, and activities like yoga or Pilates. Finding enjoyable activities and incorporating them into a regular routine is key to sustaining long-term adherence to physical activity.

c. Stress management and relaxation techniques

In today's fast-paced and demanding world, stress has become a common part of daily life. Excessive or chronic stress can have detrimental effects on both physical and mental health. Therefore, it is essential to develop effective stress management and relaxation techniques to promote overall well-being.

One widely recognized relaxation technique is deep breathing. Deep breathing exercises involve slow, deep inhalation through the nose, followed by a slow exhalation through the mouth. This practice helps activate the body's relaxation response, reducing heart rate, blood pressure, and stress hormone levels.

Mindfulness meditation is another powerful tool for stress management. It involves bringing one's attention to the present moment, without judgment or attachment to thoughts or emotions. Regular mindfulness practice has been shown to reduce stress, enhance self-awareness, improve focus and concentration, and cultivate a sense of inner calm.

Engaging in regular physical activity, as discussed earlier, is also an effective way to manage stress. Exercise helps release tension, improves mood, and promotes the production of endorphins, which are natural stress-fighting hormones.

In addition to these practices, other relaxation techniques include progressive muscle relaxation, where one systematically tenses and relaxes different muscle groups, and visualization exercises, where individuals imagine themselves in a peaceful and calming environment.

Finding healthy coping mechanisms and engaging in activities that bring joy and relaxation is also important for managing stress. This can include hobbies, spending time in nature, practicing yoga or tai chi, listening to music, journaling, or seeking support from loved ones or professionals when needed.

By incorporating stress management and relaxation techniques into daily life, individuals can reduce the negative impact of stress on their physical and mental well-being, promote a sense of balance and harmony, and enhance overall quality of life.

The Mediterranean Diet Pyramid

a. Understanding the structure and components

The Mediterranean Diet is characterized by a specific structure and components that contribute to its health-promoting properties. Understanding these elements is key to effectively adopting and following the diet.

- Plant-based emphasis: At the core of the Mediterranean Diet is a strong emphasis on plant-based foods. These include fruits, vegetables, whole grains, legumes, nuts, and seeds. These foods form the foundation of the diet and should make up a significant portion of daily meals. They provide essential vitamins, minerals, dietary fiber, and antioxidants, which support overall health and well-being.
- Healthy fats: The Mediterranean Diet encourages the consumption of healthy fats, particularly olive oil. Olive oil is a primary source of fat in the diet and is used in cooking, dressings, and marinades. It is rich in monounsaturated fats and has been associated with numerous health benefits, including heart health and reduced inflammation. Other sources of healthy fats in the Mediterranean Diet include avocados, nuts, and seeds.
- Moderate fish and poultry intake: The Mediterranean Diet includes moderate consumption of fish and poultry. Fish, especially fatty fish like salmon, mackerel, and sardines, are rich in omega-3 fatty acids, which have been linked to heart health and cognitive function. Poultry, such as chicken and turkey, can be

enjoyed in moderation as lean sources of protein.

- Limited red meat: Red meat, including beef, pork, and lamb, is consumed in smaller quantities and less frequently in the Mediterranean Diet. This is because high consumption of red meat has been associated with increased risks of certain health conditions, such as heart disease and certain types of cancer. When red meat is consumed, it is recommended to choose lean cuts and practice portion control.
- Dairy in moderation: Dairy products, such as cheese and yogurt, are consumed in moderation in the Mediterranean Diet. These products provide calcium, protein, and probiotics, but they can also be high in saturated fats. Opting for low-fat or reduced-fat varieties can help maintain a healthy balance.
- Moderate alcohol consumption: Moderate alcohol intake, typically in the form of red wine, is often associated with the Mediterranean Diet. However, it's important to note that this component is optional and should be consumed in moderation. Moderate alcohol consumption means one drink per day for women and up to two drinks per day for men.

b. Emphasizing plant-based foods

One of the distinguishing features of the Mediterranean Diet is its emphasis on plant-based foods. This dietary pattern encourages the consumption of a wide variety of fruits, vegetables, whole grains, legumes, nuts, and seeds. Plant-based foods are rich in vitamins, minerals, dietary fiber, and antioxidants, offering numerous health benefits.

- Fruits and vegetables: The Mediterranean Diet promotes the consumption of a diverse range of colorful fruits and vegetables. These foods are packed with essential nutrients, including vitamins, minerals, and antioxidants. They provide protection against chronic diseases, promote healthy digestion, support immune function, and contribute to overall vitality.
- Whole grains: Whole grains, such as whole wheat, oats, barley, quinoa, and brown rice, are integral to the Mediterranean Diet. They are high in fiber, which aids in digestion, supports heart health, and helps regulate blood sugar levels. Whole grains also provide essential nutrients, including B vitamins, iron, and magnesium.
- Legumes: Legumes, such as beans, lentils, chickpeas, and peas, are excellent sources of plant-based protein, fiber, and complex carbohydrates. They are low in fat and cholesterol, and their consumption has been associated with reduced risk of heart disease, improved blood sugar control, and weight management.
- Nuts and seeds: The Mediterranean Diet encourages the consumption of nuts and seeds, including almonds, walnuts, flaxseeds, and chia seeds. These foods are rich in healthy fats, protein, fiber, and various micronutrients. They have been linked to reduced inflammation, improved heart

health, and enhanced brain function. Incorporating these plant-based foods into meals can be done in various ways. For example, adding vegetables to salads, stir-fries, and soups; incorporating whole grains into main dishes or side dishes; including legumes in stews, curries, or salads; and using nuts and seeds as toppings or snacks.

c. Moderation of animal-based foods

While the Mediterranean Diet does include some animal-based foods, it emphasizes moderation and portion control. This approach is based on research suggesting that excessive consumption of animal-based products, particularly red meat, may be associated with increased health risks. By moderating the intake of animal-based foods, the Mediterranean Diet aims to promote a more balanced and sustainable approach to nutrition.

- Red meat: The consumption of red meat, including beef, pork, and lamb, is limited in the Mediterranean Diet. Red meat can be high in saturated fats, which, when consumed in excess, can increase the risk of heart disease and other health conditions. When choosing to include red meat, it is recommended to opt for lean cuts, trim visible fat, and practice portion control.

- Poultry: Poultry, such as chicken and turkey, is included in the Mediterranean Diet but in moderation. These lean sources of protein can be enjoyed as alternatives to red meat. It is advisable to remove the skin and choose lean cuts of poultry to reduce the intake of saturated fat.
- Fish and seafood: The Mediterranean Diet encourages the consumption of fish and seafood, which provide lean protein and are rich in omega-3 fatty acids. Omega-3 fatty acids have been linked to various health benefits, including heart health and cognitive function. Fatty fish, such as salmon, mackerel, and sardines, are particularly high in omega-3s.

By emphasizing plant-based foods and moderating the intake of animal-based foods, the Mediterranean Diet promotes a balance that is beneficial for overall health. This approach ensures an adequate intake of essential nutrients from a variety of sources while minimizing potential health risks associated with excessive consumption of animal-based products.

Key Principles of the Mediterranean Diet

a. Importance of whole, unprocessed foods

One of the fundamental principles of the Mediterranean

Diet is the emphasis on whole, unprocessed foods. Whole foods refer to foods that are as close to their natural state as possible, without being refined, processed, or stripped of their nutritional value. Here are some reasons why whole, unprocessed foods are considered important in the Mediterranean Diet:

- Nutrient density: Whole foods are rich in essential nutrients, including vitamins, minerals, and antioxidants. By consuming a variety of whole foods, individuals can ensure they are getting a wide range of nutrients that are necessary for optimal health and well-being.
- Dietary fiber: Whole foods, such as fruits, vegetables, whole grains, and legumes, are excellent sources of dietary fiber. Fiber is important for digestive health, as it aids in regular bowel movements, prevents constipation, and supports a healthy gut microbiome. It also helps promote satiety and can assist with weight management.
- Lower in additives and preservatives: Whole foods are typically free from artificial additives, preservatives, and added sugars. Consuming foods in their natural state helps reduce the intake of potentially harmful substances and supports a cleaner, more nutrient-dense diet.
- Sustained energy levels: Whole foods, particularly complex carbohydrates found in whole grains and legumes, provide a steady release of energy. They are digested more slowly, preventing rapid spikes

in blood sugar levels and promoting sustained energy throughout the day.

- Reduced intake of unhealthy fats and sugars: Many processed and refined foods contain unhealthy fats, such as trans fats, and added sugars. These can contribute to various health issues, including heart disease, obesity, and diabetes. By focusing on whole foods, individuals can reduce their intake of these harmful substances and promote better overall health.

b. Role of olive oil and healthy fats

Olive oil is a staple component of the Mediterranean Diet and is considered a healthy fat. Here's why olive oil and other healthy fats are important in the diet:

- Heart health: Olive oil is rich in monounsaturated fats, particularly oleic acid, which is known to have beneficial effects on heart health. It helps reduce levels of LDL cholesterol (the "bad" cholesterol) while increasing levels of HDL cholesterol (the "good" cholesterol), which can help protect against heart disease.
- Anti-inflammatory properties: Healthy fats, including those found in olive oil, have anti-inflammatory properties. Chronic inflammation is linked to various health conditions, including heart disease, cancer, and autoimmune disorders. By incorporating healthy fats into the diet, individuals can help reduce inflammation and promote overall well-being.

- Absorption of fat-soluble nutrients: Many essential vitamins and antioxidants are fat-soluble, meaning they need fat for proper absorption in the body. Healthy fats, such as olive oil, aid in the absorption of these nutrients, allowing the body to utilize them effectively.
- Flavor and satisfaction: Healthy fats add flavor and richness to meals, making them more satisfying and enjoyable. This can help promote a sense of satiety and prevent overeating, as individuals feel more content with their meals.

It's important to note that while healthy fats like olive oil are beneficial, moderation is key. Healthy fats are still calorie-dense, so portion control should be practiced to maintain a healthy weight.

c. Consumption of fish and seafood

The Mediterranean Diet promotes the consumption of fish and seafood as part of a balanced eating plan. Here's why fish and seafood are valued components of the diet:

- Omega-3 fatty acids: Fatty fish, such as salmon, mackerel, tuna, and sardines, are excellent sources of omega-3 fatty acids. These essential fats have been shown to have numerous health benefits, including reducing inflammation, supporting heart health, and promoting brain function.
- Protein-rich alternative: Fish and seafood are

excellent sources of lean protein. They provide essential amino acids necessary for the growth, repair, and maintenance of body tissues. Choosing fish and seafood as protein sources can be a healthier option compared to red meat, which is higher in saturated fats.

- Low in saturated fats: Fish and seafood are generally low in saturated fats, which can be harmful to heart health when consumed in excess. The Mediterranean Diet encourages the consumption of lean protein sources, and fish and seafood fit well within this framework.
- Versatility in cooking: Fish and seafood offer a wide range of culinary possibilities. They can be grilled, baked, steamed, or sautéed with various herbs, spices, and marinades, making them a versatile and flavorful addition to meals.

d. Incorporating fresh fruits and vegetables

Fresh fruits and vegetables are integral components of the Mediterranean Diet. Here's why incorporating them is important:

- Abundance of nutrients: Fruits and vegetables are packed with essential vitamins, minerals, antioxidants, and dietary fiber. They provide a wide range of nutrients necessary for optimal health, including vitamins A, C, and K, folate, potassium, and antioxidants that help protect against chronic diseases.
- Hydration and fiber: Many fruits and vegetables

- have high water content, contributing to hydration. They are also excellent sources of dietary fiber, aiding in digestion, promoting bowel regularity, and supporting a healthy weight.
- Antioxidant power: Fruits and vegetables are rich in antioxidants, which help protect the body against cellular damage caused by free radicals. Antioxidants have been associated with a reduced risk of chronic diseases, including heart disease, certain cancers, and neurodegenerative disorders.
- Versatility and variety: Fruits and vegetables offer endless possibilities in terms of flavors, textures, and colors. They can be enjoyed fresh, cooked, or incorporated into a variety of dishes, such as salads, stir-fries, soups, and smoothies. This versatility allows for a diverse and satisfying diet.

In summary, the Mediterranean Diet emphasizes the importance of whole, unprocessed foods, including fruits, vegetables, whole grains, legumes, nuts, and seeds. It recognizes the health benefits of olive oil and other healthy fats, promotes the consumption of fish and seafood for their omega-3 fatty acids and lean protein, and highlights the value of incorporating fresh fruits and vegetables for their nutrient density and antioxidant properties. By embracing these principles, individuals can adopt a nutritious and balanced eating pattern that supports overall health and well-being.

Grains and Legumes in the Mediterranean Diet

a. Exploring different types of grains

Grains are an important component of the Mediterranean Diet, providing essential nutrients and energy. While whole grains are widely recommended, the Mediterranean Diet encourages the exploration and inclusion of different types of grains. Here are some examples of grains commonly consumed in Mediterranean cuisine:

- Whole wheat: Whole wheat grains, including wheat berries, bulgur, and whole wheat flour, are rich in fiber, vitamins, and minerals. They offer a nutty flavor and a chewy texture, making them a versatile choice for salads, pilafs, and bread.
- Barley: Barley is a nutritious grain with a slightly chewy texture. It is high in dietary fiber, vitamins, and minerals, including magnesium and selenium. Barley is commonly used in soups, stews, risottos, and as a side dish.
- Quinoa: Although not traditionally Mediterranean, quinoa has gained popularity due to its nutritional value. It is a complete protein, meaning it contains all essential amino acids. Quinoa is gluten-free, rich in fiber, and provides various minerals such as iron and magnesium. It can be used as a base for salads, pilafs, or as a substitute for rice.
- Couscous: Couscous is a staple in North African

and Middle Eastern cuisine. It is made from semolina wheat and has a light, fluffy texture. Couscous is quick to prepare and serves as a versatile side dish or can be incorporated into salads or stews.

- Farro: Farro is an ancient grain with a nutty flavor and a chewy texture. It is high in fiber, protein, and various minerals. Farro can be used in salads, soups, risottos, or as a side dish.
- Millet: Millet is a gluten-free grain that is widely consumed in Mediterranean and African cuisines. It is rich in fiber, antioxidants, and minerals such as magnesium and phosphorus. Millet can be cooked and used as a base for pilafs, porridge, or added to baked goods.

Exploring these different types of grains adds variety and nutritional value to the Mediterranean Diet. Incorporating them into meals can be done through side dishes, salads, soups, or even as substitutes in traditional recipes.

b. Benefits of legumes and their versatility

Legumes, including beans, lentils, chickpeas, and peas, are nutrient-dense foods that play a significant role in the Mediterranean Diet. Here are the benefits of legumes and their versatility in cooking:

- Nutritional powerhouse: Legumes are rich in plant-based protein, dietary fiber, complex carbohydrates, vitamins, and minerals. They are particularly high in folate, iron, potassium, and magnesium. Including legumes in the diet provides a wide range of nutrients necessary for overall health.

- Heart health: Legumes are low in saturated fat and cholesterol and high in soluble fiber, which helps lower LDL cholesterol levels. Regular consumption of legumes has been associated with a reduced risk of heart disease and improved cardiovascular health.
- Blood sugar control: The high fiber content in legumes helps regulate blood sugar levels by slowing down digestion and preventing rapid spikes in blood glucose. This makes them an excellent choice for individuals with diabetes or those looking to maintain stable blood sugar levels.
- Weight management: Legumes are nutrient-dense and provide a feeling of fullness due to their high fiber and protein content. Including legumes in meals can help promote satiety, reduce overall calorie intake, and support healthy weight management.
- Versatility in cooking: Legumes are incredibly versatile and can be used in a variety of dishes. They can be added to soups, stews, salads, and casseroles. They can also be mashed and used as a base for spreads like hummus or incorporated into veggie burgers and meatless patties.
- Economic and environmental benefits: Legumes are affordable and sustainable sources of plant-based protein. They require fewer resources

and produce fewer greenhouse gas emissions compared to animal-based protein sources. Incorporating legumes into the diet can contribute to a more sustainable food system.

c. Traditional Mediterranean recipes

One of the unique aspects of the Mediterranean Diet is its rich culinary heritage. Traditional Mediterranean recipes are not only delicious but also align with the principles of the diet. Here are a few examples of traditional Mediterranean recipes:

- Greek Salad: A refreshing and colorful salad made with fresh vegetables like tomatoes, cucumbers, red onions, and bell peppers, topped with feta cheese, olives, and a drizzle of olive oil and lemon juice.
- Ratatouille: A classic French dish consisting of a medley of sautéed vegetables such as eggplant, zucchini, bell peppers, tomatoes, onions, and garlic. It is seasoned with herbs like thyme and basil, and can be enjoyed as a main course or a side dish.
- Tabouli: A Lebanese salad made with bulgur wheat, parsley, mint, tomatoes, cucumbers, and scallions, dressed with lemon juice and olive oil. It is a light and refreshing dish that can be served as a side or a main course.
- Spanish Paella: A vibrant rice dish originating from Spain, typically made with saffron-infused

rice, vegetables, and various proteins such as chicken, seafood, and sausage. It is a flavorful and hearty one-pot meal.

- Hummus: A popular Middle Eastern dip made from cooked and mashed chickpeas blended with tahini (sesame seed paste), garlic, lemon juice, and olive oil. Hummus is often enjoyed with pita bread or as a spread in sandwiches and wraps.
- Italian Caprese Salad: A simple and elegant salad made with fresh tomatoes, mozzarella cheese, basil leaves, and a drizzle of olive oil. It showcases the flavors of ripe tomatoes and creamy cheese, complemented by aromatic basil.

These traditional Mediterranean recipes showcase the use of fresh, wholesome ingredients such as vegetables, fruits, whole grains, legumes, and olive oil. They highlight the flavors and simplicity of Mediterranean cuisine while providing a wide range of nutrients and promoting a balanced diet.

The Power of Olive Oil

a. Health benefits of olive oil

Olive oil is a key component of the Mediterranean Diet and is renowned for its numerous health benefits. Here are some of the health benefits associated with the consumption of olive oil:

- Heart health: Olive oil is rich in monounsaturated fats, particularly oleic acid, which has been shown to have positive effects on heart health. It helps reduce LDL cholesterol levels (the "bad" cholesterol) and increase HDL cholesterol levels (the "good" cholesterol), thereby reducing the risk of heart disease and stroke.
- Anti-inflammatory properties: Olive oil contains natural antioxidants, such as polyphenols and vitamin E, which have anti-inflammatory properties. Chronic inflammation is linked to various diseases, including cardiovascular disease, metabolic disorders, and certain types of cancer. The anti-inflammatory compounds in olive oil can help mitigate inflammation and promote overall well-being.
- Antioxidant activity: Olive oil is rich in antioxidants that help protect the body against oxidative stress caused by free radicals. The antioxidants in olive oil, such as oleocanthal and hydroxytyrosol, have been linked to a reduced risk of chronic diseases, including certain types of cancer, neurodegenerative disorders, and age-related macular degeneration.
- Digestive health: Olive oil has a positive impact on digestive health. It has been shown to stimulate the production of bile, which aids in the digestion and absorption of nutrients. Additionally, olive oil has a mild laxative effect that can help prevent constipation and promote regularity.
- Blood sugar control: The monounsaturated fats in olive oil can help improve insulin sensitivity and regulate blood sugar levels. Including olive oil in

meals can contribute to better glycemic control, making it beneficial for individuals with diabetes or those at risk of developing diabetes.

- Weight management: Despite being calorie-dense, olive oil has been associated with weight management. The monounsaturated fats in olive oil help promote satiety and reduce cravings, leading to better portion control and a lower risk of overeating.

b. Differentiating between types of olive oil

There are different types of olive oil available, each with its own characteristics and culinary uses. Here's a breakdown of the various types:

- Extra Virgin Olive Oil: Extra virgin olive oil is the highest quality and most flavorful type of olive oil. It is made from the first pressing of olives without the use of heat or chemicals. Extra virgin olive oil has a low acidity level (less than 0.8%) and retains the natural antioxidants and phytochemicals present in olives. It is best used in salads, dressings, and as a finishing oil to drizzle over cooked dishes.
- Virgin Olive Oil: Virgin olive oil is also made from the first pressing of olives but has a slightly higher acidity level (up to 2%). It has a milder flavor compared to extra virgin olive oil. Virgin olive oil is suitable for cooking and can be used in sautéing, roasting, and baking.
- Olive Oil (Pure or Regular): Olive oil labeled as

"pure" or "regular" is a blend of refined olive oil and virgin or extra virgin olive oil. It undergoes a refining process, which removes impurities and lowers acidity. This type of olive oil has a milder flavor and is suitable for general cooking purposes, such as frying and baking.

- Light Olive Oil: Contrary to what the name implies, "light" olive oil does not refer to its caloric content but rather its lighter flavor and color. Light olive oil is a refined oil that undergoes additional processing to remove most of the flavor and color. It has a higher smoke point, making it suitable for high-heat cooking methods like frying.

It's important to note that the health benefits associated with olive oil are primarily attributed to extra virgin and virgin olive oils, as they retain the highest levels of antioxidants and beneficial compounds.

c. Cooking tips and recipes using olive oil

Olive oil is not only a healthy choice but also a versatile ingredient in cooking. Here are some cooking tips and recipe ideas to incorporate olive oil into your culinary repertoire:

- Salad dressings: Use extra virgin olive oil as the base for homemade salad dressings. Combine it with vinegar or citrus juice, herbs, and spices for a flavorful dressing that enhances the taste of fresh greens and vegetables.

- Sautéing and stir-frying: Olive oil adds a delicate flavor when used for sautéing vegetables, tofu, or lean meats. Heat the oil over medium heat and add your ingredients, stirring occasionally until cooked to your desired tenderness.
- Roasting and grilling: Drizzle vegetables, poultry, or fish with olive oil before roasting or grilling to add moisture and enhance the flavors. The oil helps achieve a crispy exterior while keeping the food tender and juicy.
- Baking: Substitute butter or vegetable oil with olive oil in baking recipes for a healthier twist. Olive oil works well in cakes, muffins, bread, and other baked goods. Use a lighter or milder olive oil variety for baking to avoid overpowering the flavors.
- Dipping and finishing: Serve a high-quality extra virgin olive oil alongside fresh bread for dipping. You can enhance the flavor by adding balsamic vinegar, herbs, or spices. Additionally, drizzle a small amount of extra virgin olive oil over cooked dishes, such as pasta, soups, and grilled meats, as a finishing touch.
- Marinating: Create flavorful marinades by combining olive oil with herbs, spices, citrus juice, and garlic. Marinating helps tenderize meats and infuse them with delicious flavors before grilling or cooking.

Incorporating olive oil into your cooking not only adds a pleasant taste but also provides the health benefits associated with the Mediterranean Diet. Experiment with different recipes and enjoy the versatility and flavors that olive oil brings to your meals.

The Mediterranean Diet and Heart Health

a. Impact on cardiovascular health

The Mediterranean Diet has long been associated with numerous cardiovascular health benefits, and olive oil plays a crucial role in this regard. The consumption of olive oil as a primary source of fat has shown positive effects on cardiovascular health. Here are some ways olive oil impacts cardiovascular health:

- Heart-healthy fats: Olive oil is rich in monounsaturated fats, particularly oleic acid, which has been found to have a beneficial impact on cardiovascular health. These healthy fats help reduce LDL cholesterol levels (the "bad" cholesterol) and increase HDL cholesterol levels (the "good" cholesterol), leading to a healthier lipid profile.
- Antioxidant properties: Olive oil contains natural antioxidants, such as polyphenols and vitamin E, which have been linked to improved cardiovascular health. These antioxidants help protect against oxidative stress, reduce inflammation, and prevent the oxidation of

LDL cholesterol, which is a key factor in the development of heart disease.

- Anti-inflammatory effects: Chronic inflammation is a significant contributor to the development of cardiovascular disease. Olive oil's anti-inflammatory properties can help mitigate inflammation in the body and reduce the risk of heart disease. The polyphenols and other bioactive compounds present in olive oil exert anti-inflammatory effects that promote overall cardiovascular health.
- Endothelial function: The inner lining of blood vessels, called the endothelium, plays a vital role in maintaining cardiovascular health. Studies have shown that olive oil improves endothelial function, making blood vessels more flexible and reducing the risk of endothelial dysfunction, a precursor to atherosclerosis and other cardiovascular conditions.

b. Reducing the risk of heart disease

The Mediterranean Diet, with its emphasis on olive oil, has been widely recognized as a heart-healthy eating pattern that can reduce the risk of heart disease. Here's how the Mediterranean Diet, including olive oil, helps in reducing the risk of heart disease:

- Lowering LDL cholesterol: The monounsaturated fats in olive oil have been shown to lower LDL cholesterol levels, which can contribute to the development of atherosclerosis and heart disease. By replacing unhealthy fats with olive oil, individuals can improve their lipid profile and reduce the risk of heart disease.

- Preventing oxidative damage: The antioxidants present in olive oil, such as polyphenols, help protect against oxidative damage, a process that can lead to the formation of plaque in arteries. The polyphenols in olive oil have been found to inhibit the oxidation of LDL cholesterol, reducing the risk of plaque formation and narrowing of blood vessels.

- Blood pressure management: High blood pressure is a significant risk factor for heart disease. The Mediterranean Diet, including olive oil, has been associated with lower blood pressure levels. The monounsaturated fats and antioxidants in olive oil contribute to improved blood vessel function and help regulate blood pressure.

- Anti-inflammatory effects: Chronic inflammation is closely linked to the development of heart disease. The Mediterranean Diet, rich in olive oil, is known for its anti-inflammatory properties. The polyphenols and other bioactive compounds in olive oil help reduce inflammation in the body, protecting against the development of cardiovascular conditions.

- Diabetes prevention: Type 2 diabetes is a risk factor for heart disease. The Mediterranean Diet, which includes olive oil as the primary source of fat, has been found to lower the risk of developing type 2 diabetes. By managing blood sugar levels and improving insulin sensitivity, olive oil can help prevent diabetes and reduce the associated cardiovascular risks.

c. Managing cholesterol levels

Olive oil is an excellent choice for managing cholesterol levels, particularly LDL cholesterol. Here's how olive oil can help in managing cholesterol levels:

- Replacing unhealthy fats: Saturated and trans fats are known to raise LDL cholesterol levels and increase the risk of heart disease. By substituting these unhealthy fats with olive oil, individuals can lower their intake of LDL-raising fats, thereby improving their cholesterol profile.
- Monounsaturated fats: Olive oil is primarily composed of monounsaturated fats, which have been found to have a positive impact on cholesterol levels. Monounsaturated fats help reduce LDL cholesterol while maintaining or increasing HDL cholesterol levels, leading to a healthier cholesterol ratio.
- Polyphenols and antioxidants: The polyphenols and antioxidants present in olive oil have been shown to prevent the oxidation of LDL cholesterol, a crucial step in the development of atherosclerosis. By inhibiting LDL oxidation, olive oil helps protect against the formation of plaque in the arteries, reducing the risk of heart disease.
- Omega-3 fatty acids: While olive oil is not a significant source of omega-3 fatty acids, it is often consumed as part of a diet that includes fish

and seafood, which are rich in these heart-healthy fats. Omega-3 fatty acids help lower triglyceride levels and reduce inflammation, contributing to overall cardiovascular health.

It's important to note that while olive oil can have positive effects on cholesterol levels, it should be consumed in moderation as part of a balanced diet. Portion control and overall calorie intake should be considered to maintain a healthy weight and manage cholesterol effectively. Consulting with a healthcare professional or registered dietitian can provide personalized guidance on incorporating olive oil into a cholesterol-lowering diet plan.

Weight Management with the Mediterranean Diet

a. Understanding the diet's role in weight loss

The Mediterranean Diet is often praised not only for its health benefits but also for its potential in supporting weight loss and weight management. While weight loss is a complex process influenced by various factors, the Mediterranean Diet can play a significant role. Here's how the diet's principles contribute to weight loss:

- Emphasis on whole, unprocessed foods: The Mediterranean Diet promotes the consumption of whole, nutrient-dense foods, such as fruits, vegetables, whole grains, legumes, nuts, and seeds. These foods tend to be lower in calories and higher in fiber, which helps increase satiety and reduce overall calorie intake, leading to weight loss.
- Healthy fats and portion control: Although the Mediterranean Diet includes fats, they primarily come from sources like olive oil, avocados, and nuts, which are rich in monounsaturated and polyunsaturated fats. These healthy fats provide satiety and flavor to meals while promoting heart health. However, it's important to practice portion control, as fats are calorie-dense.
- Plant-based focus: The Mediterranean Diet places a strong emphasis on plant-based foods, which are typically lower in calories and higher in fiber compared to animal-based foods. By prioritizing fruits, vegetables, whole grains, and legumes, individuals can reduce calorie intake while increasing nutrient density.
- Moderation of red meat and sweets: The Mediterranean Diet suggests limited consumption of red meat and sweets, which tend to be higher in calories, unhealthy fats, and added sugars. By reducing the intake of these calorie-dense foods, individuals can create a calorie deficit, leading to weight loss.
- Social and cultural aspects: The Mediterranean Diet encourages mindful eating and emphasizes the social and cultural aspects of meals. Taking

time to enjoy meals, savoring flavors, and eating in the company of others can promote a more mindful approach to eating, helping individuals tune in to hunger and fullness cues, leading to better portion control and overall calorie intake.

It's important to note that weight loss is a multifaceted journey, and individual results may vary. Combining the Mediterranean Diet with other healthy lifestyle practices, such as regular physical activity and stress management, can further support weight loss efforts.

b. Strategies for maintaining a healthy weight

Maintaining a healthy weight is as important as achieving weight loss. The Mediterranean Diet provides a sustainable approach to weight management. Here are some strategies for maintaining a healthy weight while following the Mediterranean Diet:

- Portion control: While the Mediterranean Diet promotes whole, unprocessed foods, it's still important to practice portion control. Even healthy foods can contribute to weight gain if consumed in excess. Pay attention to portion sizes and listen to your body's hunger and fullness cues.
- Mindful eating: The Mediterranean Diet encourages mindful eating, which involves paying full attention to the eating experience. Slow

down, savor the flavors, and be present during meals. This practice can help prevent overeating and promote a healthier relationship with food.

- Regular physical activity: Physical activity is a crucial component of maintaining a healthy weight. Combine the Mediterranean Diet with regular exercise to support weight management. Engage in activities you enjoy, such as walking, cycling, swimming, or dancing. Aim for at least 150 minutes of moderate-intensity aerobic activity per week, along with strength training exercises.

- Hydration: Stay hydrated by drinking plenty of water throughout the day. Sometimes, thirst can be mistaken for hunger, leading to unnecessary calorie consumption. Drinking water can help prevent this confusion and support overall weight management.

- Consistency and balance: Consistency is key when maintaining a healthy weight. Strive for consistency in your eating patterns and food choices, focusing on a balanced diet that includes a variety of fruits, vegetables, whole grains, lean proteins, and healthy fats. Avoid extreme or restrictive diets, as they are not sustainable in the long term.

- Regular monitoring: Keep track of your progress by periodically monitoring your weight and body measurements. Regular monitoring can help you identify any changes and make adjustments if needed.

c. Combining the Mediterranean Diet with exercise

Combining the Mediterranean Diet with regular physical exercise can enhance the benefits for weight management and overall health. Here's how exercise complements the Mediterranean Diet:

- Increased calorie expenditure: Exercise helps burn calories, contributing to creating a calorie deficit necessary for weight loss or weight management. By engaging in physical activity, you can increase your daily calorie expenditure and potentially achieve your weight goals more efficiently.
- Improved body composition: Exercise, particularly strength training, helps build lean muscle mass. Increasing muscle mass can boost your metabolism, as muscles require more energy (calories) to maintain than fat tissue. This can aid in weight management and contribute to a more favorable body composition.
- Enhanced cardiovascular health: The Mediterranean Diet already promotes cardiovascular health, and exercise further strengthens the cardiovascular system. Regular aerobic exercise, such as brisk walking, jogging, cycling, or swimming, can improve cardiovascular fitness, lower blood pressure, and reduce the risk of heart disease.
- Stress management: Exercise is an effective stress management tool. By engaging in physical

activity, you release endorphins, which are natural mood boosters. Regular exercise can help reduce stress levels and emotional eating, supporting weight management efforts.

- Overall well-being: The combination of the Mediterranean Diet and exercise can improve overall well-being and quality of life. Physical activity promotes better sleep, increased energy levels, and improved mental health, all of which contribute to a healthier lifestyle and sustainable weight management.

When combining the Mediterranean Diet with exercise, aim for a balanced approach. Start gradually and choose activities that you enjoy and can sustain in the long term. Consult with a healthcare professional or a certified fitness trainer to develop an exercise plan that suits your fitness level and goals. Remember to listen to your body, rest when needed, and celebrate the progress you make along the way.

Mediterranean Diet Meal Planning

a. Developing a Weekly Meal Plan

Developing a weekly meal plan is an excellent way to streamline your food choices, save time and money, and ensure you have a balanced diet throughout the week. By planning your meals in advance, you can also avoid the stress of deciding what to eat each day. Here are some steps to help you create an effective weekly meal plan.

- Assess Your Needs: Start by considering your dietary goals, preferences, and any dietary restrictions or allergies. Determine the number of meals you want to plan for each day and identify the nutrients you want to incorporate.
- Create a Template: Design a meal planning template that suits your needs. It can be a simple table with days of the week and meal categories (breakfast, lunch, dinner, and snacks), or you can use an online meal planning tool or app.
- Gather Recipes: Look for recipe ideas that align with your dietary goals and preferences. Consider including a variety of proteins, whole grains, fruits, vegetables, and healthy fats in your meals. You can explore cookbooks, websites, or even create your own recipes.
- Plan Meals: Fill in your meal plan template by assigning specific recipes or meal ideas to each day and meal category. Aim for a balance of flavors, textures, and nutrients. Don't forget to account for leftovers, as they can be utilized for subsequent meals.
- Make a Grocery List: Once you have your meals planned, create a comprehensive grocery list. Take inventory of your pantry and fridge to ensure you don't buy unnecessary items. Organize the list according to sections in the grocery store to save time.
- Shop Wisely: When grocery shopping, stick to your list and avoid impulsive purchases. Opt for

fresh, seasonal produce, and choose whole foods over processed ones. Buying in bulk and utilizing sales or coupons can also help you save money.

- Prep Ahead: To make your week go smoother, consider prepping some ingredients or meals in advance. You can chop vegetables, marinate proteins, or even cook entire meals and portion them for later use. This saves time during busy weekdays.
- Stay Flexible: While a weekly meal plan provides structure, it's important to remain flexible. If unexpected events occur or you simply don't feel like eating what you planned for a particular day, don't hesitate to make adjustments. Use your creativity to modify your meals while still meeting your nutritional needs.

Developing a weekly meal plan allows you to take control of your nutrition, eliminate decision fatigue, and reduce food waste. By incorporating a variety of ingredients, you can ensure a well-rounded diet. Experiment with different recipes and cuisines to keep your meals exciting and enjoyable.

b. Tips for Grocery Shopping and Food Preparation

Efficient grocery shopping and food preparation are essential components of maintaining a healthy and organized kitchen. With a few tips and tricks, you can streamline your shopping trips and make the most of your time in the kitchen. Here are some suggestions to help you improve your grocery shopping and food preparation routine.

- Plan Before You Shop: Before heading to the grocery store, take a few minutes to plan your meals for the upcoming week. Refer to your meal plan and create a detailed grocery list based on the recipes you intend to make. This will help you avoid impulse purchases and ensure you have all the necessary ingredients.
- Shop with a Full Stomach: Shopping while hungry can lead to impulsive purchases and unhealthy food choices. Eat a nutritious meal or snack before heading to the grocery store to make more rational decisions and stick to your list.
- Stick to the Perimeter: The perimeter of most grocery stores is where you'll find fresh produce, meats, and dairy products. These whole foods are generally healthier options compared to processed and packaged foods found in the inner aisles. Focus on filling your cart with fruits, vegetables, lean proteins, and whole grains.
- Read Labels: When buying packaged foods, it's important to read the labels carefully. Look for ingredients you recognize and understand, and avoid products high in added sugars, unhealthy fats, and artificial additives. Pay attention to serving sizes to ensure you're aware of the portion you're consuming.
- Practice Batch Cooking: Consider dedicating a

few hours each week to batch cooking. Prepare large quantities of staple ingredients like grains, proteins, and roasted vegetables, and store them in the fridge or freezer for later use. This makes it easier to assemble quick and nutritious meals during busy weekdays.

- Embrace Meal Prep Containers: Invest in a set of reusable meal prep containers. These containers allow you to portion out meals in advance, making it convenient to grab a pre-portioned meal when you're on the go or have a busy schedule. They also help with portion control.
- Use Time-Saving Kitchen Tools: Utilize kitchen tools that can help speed up food preparation. For example, a food processor can quickly chop vegetables, a blender can make smoothies or soups, and a slow cooker can simmer ingredients while you're away. These tools can save you valuable time and effort.
- Practice Proper Food Storage: Properly storing your food is crucial for maintaining its freshness and preventing foodborne illnesses. Invest in quality food storage containers that are airtight and can be easily stacked. Label and date your containers to keep track of leftovers and prevent food waste.

By implementing these tips, you can make grocery shopping and food preparation more efficient and enjoyable. With proper planning, smart shopping choices, and time-saving strategies, you'll have a well-stocked kitchen and healthy meals ready to go.

c. Sample Meal Plans

Here are three sample meal plans that provide a variety of nutritious meals for a week. These plans can serve as inspiration and be modified based on your dietary preferences and needs.

Sample Meal Plan 1:

Day 1:

- Breakfast: Greek yogurt with mixed berries and a sprinkle of granola.
- Lunch: Quinoa salad with roasted vegetables and grilled chicken.
- Snack: Carrot sticks with hummus.
- Dinner: Baked salmon with roasted sweet potatoes and steamed broccoli.
- Dessert: Fresh fruit salad.

Day 2:

- Breakfast: Spinach and mushroom omelet with whole-grain toast.
- Lunch: Chickpea and vegetable wrap with a side of mixed greens.
- Snack: Apple slices with almond butter.
- Dinner: Beef stir-fry with brown rice and stir-fried vegetables.

- Dessert: Dark chocolate squares.

Day 3:

- Breakfast: Overnight oats with sliced banana and a drizzle of honey.
- Lunch: Lentil soup with a side salad.
- Snack: Greek yogurt with a sprinkle of nuts.
- Dinner: Grilled chicken breast with quinoa and roasted Brussels sprouts.
- Dessert: Frozen yogurt with fresh berries.

Sample Meal Plan 2:

Day 1:

- Breakfast: Scrambled eggs with avocado slices and whole-grain toast.
- Lunch: Turkey and avocado wrap with a side of cherry tomatoes.
- Snack: Trail mix with dried fruit and nuts.
- Dinner: Shrimp and vegetable stir-fry with brown rice.
- Dessert: Yogurt parfait with layered berries and granola.

Day 2:

- Breakfast: Smoothie made with spinach, banana, almond milk, and a scoop of protein powder.
- Lunch: Quinoa salad with roasted chickpeas and mixed greens.
- Snack: Celery sticks with peanut butter.
- Dinner: Baked chicken breast with roasted sweet potatoes and green beans.

- Dessert: Baked apple slices with cinnamon.

Day 3:

- Breakfast: Whole-grain pancakes topped with fresh fruit and a drizzle of maple syrup.
- Lunch: Caprese salad with mozzarella cheese, tomatoes, and basil.
- Snack: Rice cakes with almond butter.
- Dinner: Grilled salmon with quinoa and steamed asparagus.
- Dessert: Chia seed pudding with sliced almonds.

Sample Meal Plan 3:

Day 1:

- Breakfast: Oatmeal with sliced peaches and a sprinkle of cinnamon.
- Lunch: Spinach and feta salad with cherry tomatoes and grilled chicken.
- Snack: Edamame pods.
- Dinner: Vegetable curry with brown rice.
- Dessert: Frozen banana slices dipped in dark chocolate.

Day 2:

- Breakfast: Veggie scramble with bell peppers, onions, and zucchini.
- Lunch: Quinoa and black bean bowl with salsa and avocado.
- Snack: Cottage cheese with fresh pineapple chunks.
- Dinner: Baked cod with quinoa and roasted

vegetables.
- Dessert: Mixed berry smoothie.

Day 3:

- Breakfast: Whole-grain toast with smashed avocado and poached eggs.
- Lunch: Greek salad with cucumber, tomatoes, olives, and grilled shrimp.
- Snack: Kale chips.
- Dinner: Lentil curry with brown rice and steamed broccoli.
- Dessert: Mango sorbet.

Feel free to adjust these sample meal plans according to your taste preferences, dietary goals, and portion sizes. They serve as a starting point to help you structure your meals throughout the week, ensuring a healthy and balanced diet.

Conclusion

a. Recap of the Mediterranean Diet's Benefits

The Mediterranean Diet is not just a diet; it is a lifestyle that promotes overall health and well-being. It is inspired by the traditional eating patterns of countries bordering the Mediterranean Sea, such as Greece, Italy, and Spain. Let's recap some of the key benefits associated with following the Mediterranean Diet.

- Heart Health: Numerous studies have shown that the Mediterranean Diet is associated with a reduced risk of heart disease. The diet emphasizes the consumption of heart-healthy foods like fruits, vegetables, whole grains, legumes, nuts, and olive oil while limiting red meat and processed foods. It also encourages moderate consumption of fish and poultry, which are excellent sources of lean protein.
- Reduced Risk of Chronic Diseases: Following the Mediterranean Diet has been linked to a lower risk of various chronic diseases, including type 2 diabetes, certain types of cancer, and neurodegenerative conditions like Alzheimer's disease. The abundance of plant-based foods, antioxidants, and healthy fats in the diet contribute to its protective effects.
- Weight Management: The Mediterranean Diet is not a strict calorie-restricted plan, but it emphasizes nutrient-dense foods that can support healthy weight management. The diet includes plenty of fiber-rich foods, which promote feelings of fullness and can help control appetite. Additionally, the diet discourages excessive consumption of sugary beverages and highly processed snacks, which can contribute to weight gain.
- Brain Health: The Mediterranean Diet has been associated with better cognitive function and a lower risk of age-related cognitive decline. The combination of antioxidants, omega-3 fatty acids

from fish, and healthy fats from olive oil and nuts may play a role in preserving brain health and reducing the risk of cognitive impairment.

- Improved Mood and Mental Well-being: Research suggests that the Mediterranean Diet may have a positive impact on mental health. The abundance of fruits, vegetables, whole grains, and healthy fats can provide essential nutrients that support brain health and neurotransmitter function. Additionally, the social and cultural aspects of the Mediterranean lifestyle, such as shared meals and a focus on leisurely dining, contribute to overall well-being.

b. Final Words of Encouragement and Guidance

Embarking on a journey towards a healthier lifestyle, such as adopting the Mediterranean Diet, is a commendable decision. As you incorporate the principles of this eating pattern into your life, remember to approach it with patience, flexibility, and enjoyment. Here are some final words of encouragement and guidance:

- Start Gradually: Implementing major dietary changes all at once can be overwhelming. Instead, start by incorporating Mediterranean-style meals a few times a week and gradually increase the frequency. This allows you to adjust your taste preferences and adapt to new cooking methods and ingredients.

- Embrace Variety: The Mediterranean Diet celebrates the abundance of fresh, whole foods. Explore the rich variety of fruits, vegetables, whole grains, legumes, herbs, and spices available to you. Experiment with different flavors, textures, and colors to make your meals exciting and satisfying.
- Enjoy Healthy Fats: The Mediterranean Diet is known for its emphasis on healthy fats, particularly those found in olive oil, nuts, and avocados. These fats provide satiety, enhance flavor, and offer numerous health benefits. However, remember that moderation is key, as healthy fats are still calorie-dense.
- Prioritize Plant Foods: Make fruits, vegetables, whole grains, and legumes the foundation of your meals. These foods provide an array of vitamins, minerals, fiber, and antioxidants essential for optimal health. Aim to fill at least half of your plate with vegetables and include fruits as a natural and nutritious dessert option.
- Enjoy Fish and Lean Protein: Fish, particularly fatty fish like salmon, trout, and sardines, are excellent sources of omega-3 fatty acids. Aim to include fish in your meals at least twice a week. For other sources of protein, opt for lean options like poultry, legumes, and nuts.
- Stay Active: Physical activity is a vital component of a healthy lifestyle. Pairing the Mediterranean Diet with regular exercise can further enhance its benefits. Find activities you enjoy and make them a regular part of your routine.
- Foster Social Connections: The Mediterranean

lifestyle places great importance on social connections and shared meals. Embrace the opportunity to gather with loved ones, enjoy meals together, and engage in meaningful conversations. This aspect of the diet can contribute to overall well-being and happiness.

Remember, adopting the Mediterranean Diet is not about strict rules or deprivation but rather about embracing a balanced, enjoyable, and sustainable way of eating. Celebrate the process and the positive changes you're making for your health.

CHAPTER TWO

Greek Salad with Grilled Chicken

Description: The Greek Salad with Grilled Chicken is a vibrant and refreshing dish that combines the flavors of the Mediterranean with tender grilled chicken. This colorful salad is packed with crisp vegetables, tangy feta cheese, and a zesty homemade dressing. It's perfect for a light and healthy lunch or dinner.

Ingredients:

- 2 boneless, skinless chicken breasts
- 4 cups mixed salad greens
- 1 cup cherry tomatoes, halved
- 1 cucumber, sliced
- 1 red bell pepper, diced
- 1/2 red onion, thinly sliced
- 1/2 cup Kalamata olives, pitted
- 1/2 cup crumbled feta cheese
- 2 tablespoons extra-virgin olive oil
- 1 tablespoon lemon juice
- 1 clove garlic, minced
- 1 teaspoon dried oregano
- Salt and pepper to taste

Instructions:

- Preheat your grill to medium-high heat. Season

the chicken breasts with salt, pepper, and half of the dried oregano.

- Grill the chicken for about 6-8 minutes per side, or until cooked through and no longer pink in the center. Remove from the grill and let it rest for a few minutes before slicing.
- In a large bowl, combine the salad greens, cherry tomatoes, cucumber, red bell pepper, red onion, Kalamata olives, and crumbled feta cheese.
- In a small bowl, whisk together the extra-virgin olive oil, lemon juice, minced garlic, remaining dried oregano, salt, and pepper. Drizzle the dressing over the salad and toss to combine.
- Divide the salad into plates and top each portion with sliced grilled chicken.
- Serve immediately and enjoy!

Nutritional Information:

Calories: 320 kcal

Protein: 30g

Fat: 17g

Carbohydrates: 15g

Fiber: 4g

Mediterranean Baked Fish

Description: The Mediterranean Baked Fish is a delightful seafood dish inspired by the flavors of the Mediterranean coast. Tender white fish fillets are baked to perfection with a medley of aromatic herbs, juicy tomatoes, briny olives, and tangy lemon. This healthy and flavorful meal is simple to prepare and will transport your taste buds to the shores of the Mediterranean.

Ingredients:

- 4 white fish fillets (such as cod, haddock, or sea bass)
- 2 tablespoons extra-virgin olive oil
- 2 cloves garlic, minced
- 1 teaspoon dried oregano
- 1/2 teaspoon dried thyme
- 1/2 teaspoon paprika
- Salt and pepper to taste
- 1 cup cherry tomatoes, halved
- 1/2 cup Kalamata olives, pitted
- 1 lemon, sliced
- Fresh parsley, chopped (for garnish)

Instructions:

- Preheat your oven to 400°F (200°C). Lightly grease a baking dish with olive oil.
- Place the fish fillets in the prepared baking dish. Drizzle them with extra-virgin olive oil and sprinkle minced garlic, dried oregano, dried thyme, paprika, salt, and pepper evenly over the fillets.
- Arrange the cherry tomatoes, Kalamata olives, and lemon slices around the fish in the baking

dish.
- Bake for 15-20 minutes, or until the fish is cooked through and flakes easily with a fork.
- Remove from the oven and garnish with fresh parsley.
- Serve the Mediterranean Baked Fish with your favorite side dishes or over a bed of couscous or quinoa.
- Enjoy the flavors of the Mediterranean!

Nutritional Information:

Calories: 250 kcal

Protein: 28g

Fat: 12g

Carbohydrates: 8g

Fiber: 2g

Vegetable and Chickpea Stew

Description: The Vegetable and Chickpea Stew is a hearty and nutritious dish filled with a colorful assortment of vegetables, tender chickpeas, and aromatic herbs. This vegetarian stew is bursting with flavors and makes a satisfying meal on its own or served with crusty bread. It's perfect for those seeking a healthy and comforting option for lunch or dinner.

Ingredients:

- 1 tablespoon olive oil
- 1 onion, chopped
- 2 cloves garlic, minced
- 1 carrot, diced
- 1 zucchini, diced
- 1 red bell pepper, diced
- 1 can (15 oz) chickpeas, drained and rinsed
- 1 can (14 oz) diced tomatoes
- 2 cups vegetable broth
- 1 teaspoon dried basil
- 1 teaspoon dried oregano
- 1/2 teaspoon paprika
- Salt and pepper to taste
- Fresh parsley, chopped (for garnish)

Instructions:

- Heat olive oil in a large pot or Dutch oven over medium heat. Add the chopped onion and minced garlic, and sauté until fragrant and translucent.
- Add the diced carrot, zucchini, and red bell pepper to the pot. Cook for a few minutes, until the vegetables start to soften.
- Stir in the chickpeas, diced tomatoes (with their juices), vegetable broth, dried basil, dried oregano, paprika, salt, and pepper.
- Bring the stew to a boil, then reduce the heat to low. Cover and simmer for 20-25 minutes, or until the vegetables are tender.
- Taste and adjust the seasoning if needed.

- Serve the Vegetable and Chickpea Stew hot, garnished with fresh parsley.
- Enjoy the comforting flavors and nourishing goodness!

Nutritional Information:

Calories: 220 kcal

Protein: 9g

Fat: 5g

Carbohydrates: 36g

Fiber: 8g

Spinach and Feta Stuffed Chicken Breast

Description: The Spinach and Feta Stuffed Chicken Breast is an elegant and flavorful dish that combines juicy chicken breast with a delightful filling of spinach and tangy feta cheese. This dish is not only visually appealing but also a healthy and satisfying option for dinner. With every bite, you'll enjoy the tender chicken and the burst of flavors from the spinach and feta stuffing.

Ingredients:

- 4 boneless, skinless chicken breasts

- 2 cups fresh spinach leaves
- 1/2 cup crumbled feta cheese
- 2 cloves garlic, minced
- 1 tablespoon olive oil
- 1 teaspoon dried basil
- 1 teaspoon dried thyme
- Salt and pepper to taste
- Toothpicks (for securing the chicken)

Instructions:

- Preheat your oven to 375°F (190°C). Grease a baking dish with olive oil or cooking spray.
- In a large skillet, heat the olive oil over medium heat. Add the minced garlic and sauté for about 1 minute, until fragrant.
- Add the fresh spinach leaves to the skillet and cook until wilted, stirring occasionally. Remove from heat and let it cool slightly.
- In a bowl, combine the wilted spinach, crumbled feta cheese, dried basil, dried thyme, salt, and pepper. Mix well.
- Using a sharp knife, cut a pocket horizontally into each chicken breast. Be careful not to cut all the way through.
- Stuff each chicken breast with the spinach and feta mixture, then secure the openings with toothpicks.
- Place the stuffed chicken breasts in the prepared baking dish. Season the outside with salt, pepper, dried basil, and dried thyme.
- Bake in the preheated oven for 25-30 minutes, or until the chicken is cooked through and no longer pink in the center.

- Remove the toothpicks before serving.
- Serve the Spinach and Feta Stuffed Chicken Breast with your favorite side dishes or a fresh salad.
- Enjoy this delightful and flavorful meal!

Nutritional Information:

Calories: 280 kcal

Protein: 42g

Fat: 10g

Carbohydrates: 4g

Fiber: 1g

Greek-Style Grilled Lamb Chops

Description: Greek-Style Grilled Lamb Chops are succulent and flavorful, marinated in a mixture of olive oil, lemon juice, garlic, and aromatic herbs. These tender lamb chops are perfect for a Mediterranean-inspired feast. Grilled to perfection, they are juicy on the inside and nicely charred on the outside, offering a delightful dining experience.

Ingredients:

- 8 lamb chops
- 3 tablespoons extra-virgin olive oil
- 2 tablespoons fresh lemon juice

- 3 cloves garlic, minced
- 1 teaspoon dried oregano
- 1 teaspoon dried rosemary
- Salt and pepper to taste

Instructions:

- In a bowl, whisk together the olive oil, lemon juice, minced garlic, dried oregano, dried rosemary, salt, and pepper.
- Place the lamb chops in a shallow dish or zip-top bag. Pour the marinade over the chops, making sure they are well coated. Marinate in the refrigerator for at least 2 hours, or overnight for maximum flavor.
- Preheat your grill to medium-high heat. Remove the lamb chops from the marinade and discard the excess marinade.
- Grill the lamb chops for about 4-6 minutes per side, depending on your desired level of doneness. For medium-rare, aim for an internal temperature of 145°F (63°C).
- Remove the lamb chops from the grill and let them rest for a few minutes before serving.
- Serve the Greek-Style Grilled Lamb Chops with a side of roasted potatoes, Greek salad, or grilled vegetables.
- Enjoy the rich and aromatic flavors of this delicious dish!

Nutritional Information:

Calories: 380 kcal

Protein: 34g

Fat: 26g

Carbohydrates: 1g

Fiber: 0g

Mediterranean Quinoa Salad

Description: The Mediterranean Quinoa Salad is a vibrant and nutritious dish that combines fluffy quinoa with a medley of fresh vegetables, tangy olives, and creamy feta cheese. Dressed with a zesty lemon and olive oil dressing, this salad is bursting with Mediterranean flavors and makes a perfect side dish or light lunch option.

Ingredients:

- 1 cup cooked quinoa, cooled
- 1 cup cherry tomatoes, halved
- 1 cucumber, diced
- 1 red bell pepper, diced
- 1/4 cup red onion, finely chopped
- 1/4 cup Kalamata olives, pitted and halved
- 1/4 cup crumbled feta cheese
- 2 tablespoons fresh lemon juice
- 2 tablespoons extra-virgin olive oil
- 1 clove garlic, minced
- 1 teaspoon dried oregano

- Salt and pepper to taste
- Fresh parsley, chopped (for garnish)

Instructions:

- In a large bowl, combine the cooked quinoa, cherry tomatoes, diced cucumber, diced red bell pepper, chopped red onion, Kalamata olives, and crumbled feta cheese.
- In a small bowl, whisk together the fresh lemon juice, extra-virgin olive oil, minced garlic, dried oregano, salt, and pepper.
- Drizzle the dressing over the quinoa salad and toss gently to combine.
- Let the salad sit for about 10 minutes to allow the flavors to meld together.
- Garnish with fresh parsley before serving.
- Serve the Mediterranean Quinoa Salad as a side dish with grilled chicken, fish, or lamb, or enjoy it as a light and refreshing lunch on its own.
- Savor the Mediterranean-inspired goodness!

Nutritional Information:

Calories: 240 kcal

Protein: 7g

Fat: 13g

Carbohydrates: 26g

Fiber: 4g

Grilled Shrimp Skewers with Tzatziki Sauce

Description: Grilled Shrimp Skewers with Tzatziki Sauce are a delectable and healthy seafood delight. Succulent shrimp are marinated in a garlic and herb mixture, then grilled to perfection. Served with a cool and tangy tzatziki sauce, these skewers make a fantastic appetizer or main course option for any occasion.

Ingredients:

- 1 pound large shrimp, peeled and deveined
- 2 tablespoons olive oil
- 2 cloves garlic, minced
- 1 teaspoon dried dill
- 1 teaspoon dried oregano
- Salt and pepper to taste
- Wooden skewers, soaked in water for 30 minutes
- For the Tzatziki Sauce:

- 1 cup Greek yogurt
- 1/2 cucumber, grated and squeezed to remove excess moisture
- 1 clove garlic, minced
- 1 tablespoon fresh lemon juice
- 1 tablespoon extra-virgin olive oil
- 1 tablespoon fresh dill, chopped
- Salt and pepper to taste

Instructions:

- In a bowl, combine the olive oil, minced garlic, dried dill, dried oregano, salt, and pepper. Add the shrimp and toss to coat them evenly in the marinade. Let the shrimp marinate for about 20 minutes.
- Preheat your grill to medium-high heat.
- Thread the marinated shrimp onto the soaked wooden skewers, dividing them evenly.
- Place the shrimp skewers on the preheated grill and cook for about 2-3 minutes per side, until they turn pink and opaque.
- Remove the shrimp skewers from the grill and set them aside.
- In a separate bowl, prepare the tzatziki sauce by combining the Greek yogurt, grated cucumber, minced garlic, fresh lemon juice, extra-virgin olive oil, fresh dill, salt, and pepper. Mix well.
- Serve the Grilled Shrimp Skewers with the tzatziki sauce on the side.
- Enjoy these flavorful and juicy shrimp skewers as a tasty appetizer or as a main course with a side of Mediterranean salad or grilled vegetables.

Nutritional Information:

Calories: 220 kcal

Protein: 26g

Fat: 11g

Carbohydrates: 6g

Fiber: 1g

Caprese Stuffed Portobello Mushrooms

Description: Caprese Stuffed Portobello Mushrooms are a mouthwatering vegetarian delight that brings together the classic flavors of Caprese salad and combines them with savory portobello mushrooms. Stuffed with a mixture of fresh tomatoes, basil, mozzarella cheese, and balsamic glaze, these mushrooms are baked to perfection, resulting in a flavorful and satisfying dish.

Ingredients:

- 4 large portobello mushrooms
- 2 tablespoons extra-virgin olive oil
- 2 cloves garlic, minced
- 2 medium tomatoes, diced
- 1 cup fresh mozzarella cheese, diced
- 1/4 cup fresh basil leaves, chopped
- Balsamic glaze, for drizzling
- Salt and pepper to taste

Instructions:

- Preheat your oven to 375°F (190°C). Grease a baking dish with olive oil or cooking spray.
- Remove the stems from the portobello mushrooms and gently scrape out the gills using a spoon.
- In a skillet, heat the olive oil over medium heat. Add the minced garlic and sauté for about 1

minute, until fragrant.

- Add the diced tomatoes to the skillet and cook for a few minutes until slightly softened. Remove from heat and let it cool slightly.
- In a bowl, combine the cooked tomatoes, diced mozzarella cheese, chopped basil leaves, salt, and pepper.
- Place the portobello mushrooms on the prepared baking dish. Fill each mushroom cap with the tomato and mozzarella mixture.
- Bake in the preheated oven for 15-20 minutes, or until the mushrooms are tender and the cheese is melted and bubbly.
- Remove from the oven and drizzle the Caprese Stuffed Portobello Mushrooms with balsamic glaze.
- Serve as a delicious appetizer or as a main course with a side salad or crusty bread.
- Enjoy the delightful flavors and textures of this vegetarian masterpiece!

Nutritional Information:

Calories: 180 kcal

Protein: 11g

Fat: 12g

Carbohydrates: 10g

Fiber: 3g

Mediterranean Veggie Wrap

Description: This Mediterranean Veggie Wrap is a refreshing and healthy option for a quick meal. Packed with vibrant flavors and nutritious ingredients, it's perfect for a light lunch or a satisfying dinner.

Ingredients:

- 1 whole wheat tortilla
- 1/2 cup mixed salad greens
- 1/4 cup diced cucumbers
- 1/4 cup sliced bell peppers
- 1/4 cup cherry tomatoes, halved
- 2 tablespoons crumbled feta cheese
- 1 tablespoon chopped Kalamata olives
- 1 tablespoon chopped fresh parsley
- 2 tablespoons hummus
- Juice of 1/2 lemon
- Salt and pepper to taste

Instructions:

- Lay the whole wheat tortilla flat on a clean surface.
- Spread the hummus evenly over the tortilla.
- In a small bowl, combine the salad greens, cucumbers, bell peppers, cherry tomatoes, feta cheese, Kalamata olives, and parsley. Toss gently to mix.
- Place the mixed salad greens and vegetables on top

of the tortilla, leaving a border around the edges.
- Drizzle the lemon juice over the vegetables and season with salt and pepper.
- Roll the tortilla tightly, tucking in the sides as you go.
- Cut the wrap in half diagonally and serve.

Nutritional Information:

Calories: 280

Protein: 10g

Carbohydrates: 35g

Fat: 11g

Fiber: 7g

Lemon Herb Roasted Chicken

Description: The Lemon Herb Roasted Chicken is a delightful and aromatic dish that will tantalize your taste buds. The chicken is marinated in a zesty lemon and herb mixture, resulting in tender and flavorful meat. This recipe is perfect for a special dinner or any occasion that calls for a delicious roasted chicken.

Ingredients:

- 1 whole chicken (about 3-4 pounds)

- 2 lemons, juiced and zested
- 4 cloves of garlic, minced
- 2 tablespoons fresh rosemary, chopped
- 2 tablespoons fresh thyme, chopped
- 2 tablespoons olive oil
- Salt and pepper to taste

Instructions:

- Preheat the oven to 375°F (190°C).
- Rinse the whole chicken under cold water and pat it dry with paper towels.
- In a small bowl, combine the lemon juice, lemon zest, minced garlic, chopped rosemary, chopped thyme, olive oil, salt, and pepper. Mix well.
- Place the chicken in a roasting pan and generously rub the lemon herb mixture all over the chicken, making sure to get under the skin.
- Tie the legs together with kitchen twine and tuck the wings under the chicken.
- Roast the chicken in the preheated oven for about 1 hour and 30 minutes, or until the internal temperature reaches 165°F (74°C) and the skin is golden brown and crispy.
- Remove the chicken from the oven and let it rest for 10 minutes before carving.
- Serve the Lemon Herb Roasted Chicken with your favorite sides or vegetables.

Nutritional Information:

Calories: 320

Protein: 30g

Carbohydrates: 2g

Fat: 20g

Fiber: 0g

Greek Lemon Potatoes with Grilled Halloumi

Description: Greek Lemon Potatoes with Grilled Halloumi is a mouthwatering combination of tender roasted potatoes and savory grilled halloumi cheese. The potatoes are tossed in a lemon and herb dressing, creating a tangy and aromatic flavor profile. With the addition of grilled halloumi, this dish becomes a satisfying vegetarian main course or a flavorful side dish.

Ingredients:

- 4 large potatoes, peeled and cut into wedges
- Juice of 2 lemons
- 3 tablespoons olive oil
- 2 cloves of garlic, minced
- 1 teaspoon dried oregano
- Salt and pepper to taste
- 8 ounces halloumi cheese, sliced

Instructions:

- Preheat the oven to 400°F (200°C).
- In a large bowl, combine the lemon juice, olive

oil, minced garlic, dried oregano, salt, and pepper. Whisk well to emulsify the dressing.

- Add the potato wedges to the bowl and toss them in the dressing until they are evenly coated.
- Transfer the potatoes to a baking dish and spread them out in a single layer.
- Roast the potatoes in the preheated oven for about 40-45 minutes, or until they are golden brown and crispy.
- While the potatoes are roasting, heat a grill pan over medium-high heat.
- Grill the halloumi slices for 2-3 minutes on each side until they develop grill marks.
- Once the potatoes are done, remove them from the oven and let them cool slightly.
- Arrange the grilled halloumi slices on top of the roasted potatoes.
- Serve the Greek Lemon Potatoes with Grilled Halloumi as a main course or side dish.

Nutritional Information:

Calories: 380

Protein: 18g

Carbohydrates: 35g

Fat: 20g

Fiber: 4g

Tomato and Mozzarella Caprese Salad

Description: The Tomato and Mozzarella Caprese Salad is a classic Italian dish that showcases the vibrant flavors of ripe tomatoes, creamy mozzarella cheese, and fresh basil. This light and refreshing salad is perfect for hot summer days or as a side dish to accompany your favorite Italian meals.

Ingredients:

- 2 large tomatoes, sliced
- 8 ounces fresh mozzarella cheese, sliced
- Handful of fresh basil leaves
- 2 tablespoons extra virgin olive oil
- 1 tablespoon balsamic vinegar
- Salt and pepper to taste

Instructions:

- Arrange the tomato slices on a serving platter.
- Place a slice of fresh mozzarella on top of each tomato slice.
- Tuck the fresh basil leaves in between the tomato and mozzarella slices.
- Drizzle the extra virgin olive oil and balsamic vinegar over the salad.
- Sprinkle with salt and pepper to taste.
- Let the flavors meld together for a few minutes before serving.

Nutritional Information:

Calories: 240

Protein: 15g

Carbohydrates: 6g

Fat: 18g

Fiber: 2g

Mediterranean Tuna Salad

Description: The Mediterranean Tuna Salad is a light and flavorful dish that combines the freshness of mixed greens, the heartiness of tuna, and the tanginess of Mediterranean flavors. This salad is packed with protein and essential nutrients, making it a satisfying and nutritious option for a quick lunch or dinner.

Ingredients:

- 1 can (5 ounces) tuna, drained
- 2 cups mixed salad greens
- 1/4 cup diced cucumbers
- 1/4 cup sliced cherry tomatoes
- 1/4 cup sliced red onions
- 2 tablespoons Kalamata olives, pitted and halved
- 2 tablespoons crumbled feta cheese

- 1 tablespoon chopped fresh parsley
- 1 tablespoon lemon juice
- 1 tablespoon extra virgin olive oil
- Salt and pepper to taste

Instructions:

- In a large bowl, flake the tuna with a fork.
- Add the mixed salad greens, diced cucumbers, sliced cherry tomatoes, sliced red onions, Kalamata olives, crumbled feta cheese, and chopped fresh parsley to the bowl.
- Drizzle the lemon juice and extra virgin olive oil over the salad.
- Season with salt and pepper to taste.
- Toss the salad gently until all the ingredients are well combined.
- Serve the Mediterranean Tuna Salad as a refreshing and nutritious meal.

Nutritional Information:

Calories: 250

Protein: 20g

Carbohydrates: 10g

Fat: 15g

Fiber: 3g

Falafel with Tahini Sauce and Pita Bread

Description: Falafel with Tahini Sauce and Pita Bread is a popular Middle Eastern dish known for its fragrant and flavorful falafel balls. These crispy chickpea fritters are served in warm pita bread and drizzled with creamy tahini sauce. This vegetarian delight is perfect as a main course or as part of a mezze platter.

Ingredients:

- 1 cup dried chickpeas, soaked overnight
- 1/2 cup fresh parsley, chopped
- 1/2 cup fresh cilantro, chopped
- 1 small onion, chopped
- 4 cloves of garlic, minced
- 1 teaspoon ground cumin
- 1 teaspoon ground coriander
- 1/2 teaspoon baking powder
- Salt and pepper to taste
- Vegetable oil for frying
- Pita bread
- Tahini sauce (store-bought or homemade)

Instructions:

- Drain and rinse the soaked chickpeas, then transfer them to a food processor.
- Add the chopped parsley, chopped cilantro, chopped onion, minced garlic, ground cumin, ground coriander, baking powder, salt, and pepper to the food processor.
- Pulse the mixture until it becomes a coarse paste.
- Transfer the falafel mixture to a bowl, cover, and

- refrigerate for at least 1 hour to firm up.
- Heat vegetable oil in a deep pan or skillet over medium heat.
- Shape the falafel mixture into small balls or patties, approximately 1-2 inches in diameter.
- Carefully place the falafel into the hot oil and fry until golden brown and crispy, about 3-4 minutes per side.
- Remove the falafel from the oil and drain on paper towels.
- Warm the pita bread in a toaster or oven.
- Cut the pita bread in half and open the pocket.
- Stuff the pita bread with falafel balls and drizzle with tahini sauce.
- Serve the Falafel with Tahini Sauce and Pita Bread as a delicious and satisfying meal.

Nutritional Information:

Calories: 320

Protein: 10g

Carbohydrates: 45g

Fat: 12g

Fiber: 7g

Eggplant Parmesan with Whole Wheat Pasta

Description: Eggplant Parmesan with Whole Wheat Pasta

is a comforting and hearty Italian dish that combines tender slices of eggplant, tangy tomato sauce, melted cheese, and wholesome whole wheat pasta. This vegetarian recipe is perfect for a family dinner or a weekend indulgence.

Ingredients:

- 1 large eggplant, sliced into rounds
- Salt for sprinkling
- 1 cup whole wheat pasta
- 2 cups marinara sauce (store-bought or homemade)
- 1 cup shredded mozzarella cheese
- 1/2 cup grated Parmesan cheese
- Fresh basil leaves for garnish

Instructions:

- Sprinkle salt on both sides of the eggplant slices and let them sit for about 30 minutes. This helps to draw out excess moisture.
- Preheat the oven to 375°F (190°C).
- Rinse the salted eggplant slices and pat them dry with paper towels.
- Heat a grill pan or skillet over medium heat.
- Grill the eggplant slices for 2-3 minutes on each side until they develop grill marks.
- Cook the whole wheat pasta according to package instructions until al dente. Drain and set aside.
- In a baking dish, spread a thin layer of marinara sauce.

- Place a single layer of grilled eggplant slices on top of the sauce.
- Sprinkle shredded mozzarella and grated Parmesan cheese over the eggplant.
- Repeat the layers until all the ingredients are used, finishing with a layer of cheese on top.
- Cover the baking dish with foil and bake in the preheated oven for 25 minutes.
- Remove the foil and bake for an additional 10 minutes, or until the cheese is golden and bubbly.
- Remove from the oven and let it cool slightly before serving.
- Garnish with fresh basil leaves.
- Serve the Eggplant Parmesan with Whole Wheat Pasta for a satisfying and flavorful meal.

Nutritional Information:

Calories: 380

Protein: 20g

Carbohydrates: 40g

Fat: 15g

Fiber: 10g

CONCLUSION

In conclusion, the Mediterranean diet stands as a beacon of hope in our modern world, offering a pathway to improved health and overall well-being. Its emphasis on wholesome, nutrient-rich foods and balanced eating habits has proven to be a sustainable and enjoyable approach to nourishing both the body and the mind. By embracing the Mediterranean diet, we not only embrace a rich culinary tradition but also foster a profound connection with the natural world and the communities that have cultivated this way of life for centuries. As we turn the final page of this book, let us carry forward the wisdom and benefits of the Mediterranean diet, forging a path toward a healthier future for ourselves, our loved ones, and the planet we call home.

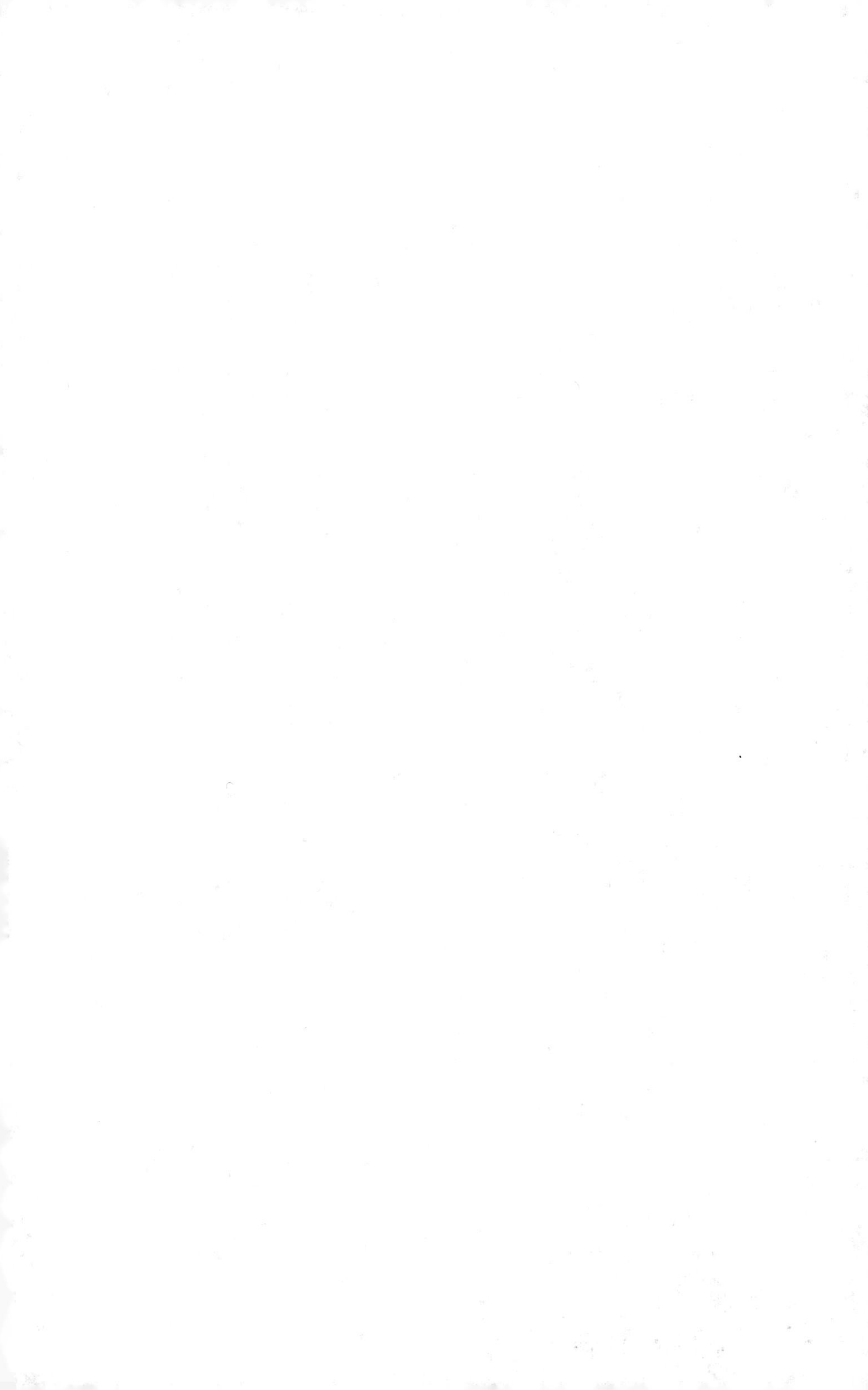

www.ingramcontent.com/pod-product-compliance
Lightning Source LLC
Chambersburg PA
CBHW050743260726
48661CB00001B/384